Table of Contents

PREVIEW 4

LYMPHOMA DIET RECIPES 7

BREAKFAST 7

1. Freezer Burritos 7

2. Banana Cookies 10

3. Savory Muffins 13

4. Egg-in-a-Hole: A Classic Idea 16

5. Egg Muffins 17

6. Frozen Sandwiches 19

7. Crockpot Casserole with Bacon and Gruyere Cheese 22

8. Banana Cake 25

9. Zucchini Chocolate Chip Cake 28

10. Blueberry Crumble Cake 31

LUNCH 34

11. Hash Brown Casserole 34

12. Make Ahead Wraps 38

13. Turkey Pesto Panini 40

14. Parmesan Crusted Tilapia 42

15. Protein Bowl 45

16. Baked Penne Pasta.. 47

17. Slow Cooker Balsamic Shredded Beef............................ 50

18. Chicken Parmesan Casserole 53

19. Oven Roasted Pork Tenderloin with Dry Rub 55

20. Ham and Cheese Sliders 57

DINNER... 59

21. Totally Tasty Taco Bar.. 59

22. Bread Machine Rolls.. 63

23. Chicken, Broccoli, and Rice Foil Packets 65

24. Chicken Parmesan Casserole.. 68

25. Baked Meatballs with Sneaky Veggies............................ 70

26. Mediterranean Shrimp 73

27. Butter Noodles 75

28. Slow Cooker Short Ribs.. 76

29. Stromboli Pizza.. 79

30. Chicken and Steak Fajitas.. 82

Lymphoma is a type of blood cancer that affects white blood cells called lymphocytes. It is also called a cancer of the lymphatic system, as it starts in the lymph glands Open a glossary item or other organs of the lymphatic system Open a glossary item.

There are 2 main types of lymphoma. These are called Hodgkin lymphoma and Non-Hodgkin lymphoma (NHL). The treatment you need depends on the type you have.

When you're looking for information about lymphoma, its important to know which type you want to know about. Ask your doctor or specialist nurse if you aren't sure.

Non-Hodgkin lymphoma accounts for approximately 85% of all lymphoma diagnoses and is the most common type of blood cancer in New Zealand.

There are many different sub types of non-Hodgkin lymphoma which are divided into 'B-cell' or 'T-cell' lymphomas. Both sup-types are cancers of the lymphatic system after the B or T lymphocytes (type of white blood cell) undergo a malignant change and multiple uncontrollably. These abnormal cells eventually form as tumours, most commonly in the lymph nodes of the body.

Hodgkin lymphoma is a rare cancer accounting for approximately 0.5% of all cancers diagnosed in New Zealand. While non-Hodgkin lymphoma can affect either the B or T cells, Hodgkin lymphoma is marked by the presence of Reed-Sternberg cells. Reed-Sternberg cells are malignant, mature B cells, and are unusually large.

Lymphoma is a cancer that occurs in white blood cells called lymphocytes. Lymphocytes help the body fight off disease. They travel through the lymphatic system, a network of lymph nodes connected by vessels. They are also located in the blood stream, bone marrow, and other organs such as the spleen.

Lymphoma develops when immature lymphocytes start multiplying rapidly due to a genetic mutation or other alteration in their biology. This can lead to tumors in the lymph nodes or other organs.

There are two main types of lymphoma: non-Hodgkin lymphoma and Hodgkin lymphoma. But within these two broad categories, there are many additional subtypes. At this time, scientists have identified more than 90 different subtypes of lymphoma.

Both Hodgkin and non-Hodgkin lymphomas can occur in children and adults, and prognosis and treatment depend on the stage and the type of cancer.

1. Freezer Burritos

Prep Time: 30 Minutes

Cook Time: 15 Minutes

Servings: 8

Ingredients

- 12 large eggs
- 1/2 cup milk (your choice)
- 1 teaspoon salt
- 1/2 ground black pepper
- 1 1/2 tablespoons butter
- 2 cups shredded Cheddar cheese
- 1 pound shredded or diced hash brown potatoes, cooked according to package directions
- 1 pound diced bacon, cooked
- 8 burrito-size tortillas
- Optional Add-Ins: sautéed veggies (bell peppers, onions, mushrooms, spinach, sweet potato), salsa,

sliced green onions, other kinds of cheeses (Monterey Jack, feta, etc)

Instructions

Make It Now:

1. Preheat the oven to 350°F.
2. In a large mixing bowl, whisk together the eggs, milk, salt, and pepper.
3. In a large skillet, melt the butter over medium heat, making sure it doesn't brown. Pour in the egg mixture and scramble the eggs until set but still moist. Remove from the heat and set aside.
4. Prepare an assembly line with all the ingredients, including 8 square pieces of foil. Assemble each burrito on top of the foil by placing approximately 1/2 cup eggs, 1/4 cup cheese, 1/3 cup potatoes, and 2 tablespoons bacon (and any additional add-ins, if desired) in the middle of the tortilla. Use a spoon or your hands to toss the ingredients before wrapping the tortilla.
5. Fold in the sides of the tortilla. While holding those in place, fold up the bottom of the tortilla over the ingredients and roll tightly into a burrito. Then, wrap

the burrito tightly in the foil. (Freezing instructions begin here.)

6. Bake for 10-15 minutes, until warmed through and the cheese is melty.

7. Freeze for Later: Follow steps 1-5. Place foil-wrapped burritos in a freezer bag, seal, and freeze.

8. Prepare From Frozen: You have three options to reheat the frozen breakfast burritos:

    1) Microwave Method: Unwrap the foil from the frozen burrito, wrap in a moist paper towel, and microwave using the defrost setting for 2 to 3 minutes, or until warmed through.

    2) Oven Method (Frozen): Preheat the oven to 350°F. Bake for 45-60 minutes, until warmed through.

    3) Oven Method (Thawed): Thaw the burritos in the refrigerator. Bake as directed in step 6.

Prep Time: 10 Minutes

Cook Time: 15 Minutes

Servings: 15

Ingredients

- 2 large ripe bananas
- 1/2 cup peanut butter, chunky or regular (sub: almond butter)
- 1/4 cup brown sugar (sub: coconut sugar for a little healthier version)
- 1/4 cup honey
- 1 teaspoon vanilla
- 1 cup rolled oats
- 1/2 cup white whole wheat flour (sub: half all-purpose and half whole wheat flour)
- 1/4 cup ground flaxseed
- 1/4 cup unsweetened protein powder (sub: almond flour, milk powder, or more white wheat flour)
- 1/4 teaspoon baking soda
- 2 teaspoons ground cinnamon

- 1/2 cup dark or semi-sweet chocolate chips (sub: carob nibs)

Instructions

Make It Now:

1. Preheat oven to 350°F.
2. Line two baking sheets with parchment paper and set aside.
3. In a large bowl, use a fork (or two forks) to mash the bananas. Then, stir together the banana, peanut butter, brown sugar, honey, and vanilla.
4. In a small bowl, combine oats, flour, flaxseed, protein powder, baking soda, and cinnamon.
5. Add the oat mixture into the banana mixture and stir until mostly combined. Add the chocolate chips and stir just until combined (do not overmix).
6. Using a cookie scoop or tablespoon, drop heaping tablespoon-sized mounds of dough roughly 2 inches apart onto prepared baking sheets. Flatten and spread the cookie dough out a bit, if you want.
7. Bake for 12-14 minutes or until browned. To store, cool completely and place in an airtight container in the fridge for 3-5 days or follow freezing directions below.

8. Freeze for Later: Cool completely and freeze in an airtight container/freezer bag for up to 2 months. Squeeze out as much air as possible.

9. Prepare From Frozen: Thaw in the fridge, on the counter, or using the defrost setting on the microwave.

Prep Time: 5 Minutes

Cook Time: 25 Minutes

Servings: 24

Ingredients

Cooking spray

- 1–2 tablespoons olive oil or avocado oil
- 1 medium-sized green or red pepper, finely chopped
- 1/2 medium-sized onion, finely chopped
- 2 cups Bisquick (all-purpose baking mix)
- 1 cup cornmeal
- 1/2 teaspoon salt
- 1/4 teaspoon pepper
- 1/4 teaspoon garlic powder
- 3 eggs
- 1 1/2 cups buttermilk
- 5 tablespoons melted butter (Can you freeze butter? Yes! Here's how.)
- 1/2 lb cooked, drained, and crumbled breakfast sausage OR 1 cup chopped cooked ham (or more if you want!)

- 2 cups shredded cheddar cheese

Instructions

Make It Now:

1. Preheat oven to 375°F. Spray two over-sized muffin tins or one regular muffin tin with cooking spray and set aside.
2. Heat the oil in a medium-sized saute pan over medium-high heat until shimmery. Saute the onion and peppers for 4-5 minutes, until softened. Set aside.
3. In a large bowl, whisk together the baking mix, cornmeal, salt, pepper, and garlic powder.
4. In another bowl, whisk together eggs, buttermilk, and butter. Stir in the sausage or ham, bell pepper, onion, and cheese to this wet mixture until combined.
5. Make a well in the middle of the dry ingredients. Pour the wet mixture into the dry mixture and stir just until combined (do not over mix).
6. Spoon the batter into the prepared muffin tins, filling three-fourths of the way up.
7. Bake for 15-20 minutes. Muffins are done when an inserted toothpick comes out clean.

8. Allow to cool in pans for a couple of minutes and then turn out onto a cooling rack.

9. Freeze for Later: Bake and let the muffins cool completely. Then place in a single layer in a gallon-sized freezer bag. Squeeze out excess air and seal. Freeze for up to 3 months.

10. Prepare From Frozen: Wrap an individual frozen muffin in a moist paper towel. Microwave on high for 30-second increments until warmed through (usually about 1 1/2 minutes total).

Prep Time: 3 Minutes

Cook Time: 5 Minutes

Servings: 4

Ingredients

- Softened butter
- Eggs
- Whole wheat bread
- Salt & pepper to taste

Instructions

1. Using a biscuit cutter, remove a circle out of the middle of a piece of bread and set it aside.
2. Generously butter one side of the bread.
3. Warm 1-2 tablespoons of butter in a skillet. (The more the better!)
4. Place bread on skillet, butter side up.
5. Crack an egg into the middle of the circle.
6. Sprinkle with salt and pepper and let it cook a few minutes on each side.

5. Egg Muffins

Prep Time: 10 Minutes

Cook Time: 18 Minutes

Servings: 12

Ingredients

- 3–4 pieces whole wheat bread, torn into small pieces (enough to fill muffin tins almost to top)
- 3–4 slices deli ham (look for preservative-free), chopped into bite-sized pieces
- 1 cup shredded cheddar cheese
- 8 large eggs
- 1 cup milk
- 2 teaspoons ground mustard
- 1/2 teaspoon ground pepper (or more or less to taste)
- Dried parsley, for garnish

Instructions

Make It Now:

1. Preheat oven to 400°F. Grease a muffin tin very well or use a silicone muffin tin.

2. Drop bread pieces evenly in muffin tins until they come about 2/3 of the way up the tin.

3. Sprinkle ham pieces evenly in each tin.

4. Sprinkle cheese evenly in each tin.

5. Whisk together eggs, milk, ground mustard, and pepper.

6. Pour egg mixture evenly in each muffin tin.

7. Sprinkle a little dried parsley on the top of each one to add a pop of color.

8. Bake for 15-18 minutes or until golden brown on top and cooked through the middle.

9. Freeze for Later: Bake according to instructions and let fully cool. Place muffins in a single layer in a gallon-sized freezer container or bag. Seal well, squeezing out excess air, and freeze.

10. Prepare From Frozen: Wrap a muffin in a moist paper towel and microwave in 30 seconds increments until heated through (about 1-2 minutes). Or thaw in the refrigerator and warm in the microwave.

Prep Time: 5 Minutes

Cook Time: 15 Minutes

Servings: 9

Ingredients

- 9 whole wheat English muffins
- 4–5 tablespoons butter, softened (optional)
- Cooking spray
- 8 large eggs
- 1/2 cup milk (your choice of milk)
- 1/2 teaspoon of salt
- 1/4 teaspoon pepper
- 9 slices Cheddar cheese (sub: Havarti, Colby-Jack, or Swiss cheese slices)
- 1 pound fully cooked bacon (try this no-fail method to bake bacon)

Instructions

Make It Now:

1. Toast English Muffins: Adjust the top oven rack to 6 inches below the broiler. Turn the broiler on high. Set the English muffins on a sheet pan and open them up with the insides facing up. Spread a little softened butter on the insides (optional). Toast under the broiler for 1-2 minutes, just until toasted. Keep a close eye on them.

2. Bake Eggs: Turn off the broiler and preheat the oven to 400°F. Spray a 9×9 inch casserole dish with cooking spray. In a mixing bowl, whisk the eggs, milk, salt, and pepper. Pour the mixture into the casserole dish. Place the casserole dish on the middle oven rack. Bake the eggs for 20 minutes, or until set in the middle. Let cool slightly and slice into 9 equal squares.

3. Assemble Sandwiches: Top each muffin bottom with one egg square, one cheese slice, and 1-2 slices of bacon that have been broken in half. Place the muffin top on and wrap the sandwich tightly in foil. (Freezing instructions begin here.)

4. Warm Sandwiches: If eating immediately, warm the foil-wrapped sandwiches in a 350°F oven for about 5 minutes, or microwave uncovered (no foil!) for 30 seconds, until cheese is melted.

5. Freeze for Later: Follow directions through Step 3. Place the individually-wrapped sandwiches in a gallon-sized freezer bag and freeze.

6. Prepare From Frozen: There are three options for warming these sandwiches.

7. Option 1 (preferred method): Thaw in refrigerator for 24 hours. Remove foil and wrap in a moist paper towel. Microwave in 30 second intervals, until warmed through (about 1-2 minutes).

8. Option 2: From frozen, remove foil and wrap frozen sandwich in a moist paper towel. Microwave for 1 minute and then in 30 second intervals, until warmed through.

9. Option 3: From frozen, place foil-wrapped sandwiches in 350° F oven for about 30 minutes or until warmed through.

Prep Time: 30 Minutes

Cook Time: 4hrs 3 Minutes

Servings: 10

Ingredients

- 1 pound (16 ounces) bacon, diced
- 1 medium yellow onion, diced (about 1 1/4 cups)
- Pinch of red pepper flakes
- 2 garlic cloves, minced
- 1 (12-ounce) jar roasted red peppers, thoroughly drained and diced (Sub: 1–2 diced red bell peppers, sautéed)
- 2 cups finely chopped kale (be sure to remove the tough stems) (Sub: spinach)
- Salt and ground black pepper, to taste

Cooking spray

- 3 cups (about 15 ounces) refrigerated or frozen shredded hash browns, thawed (it's important to thaw them first!)

- 1/2 cup shredded Parmesan cheese (sub: grated Parmesan cheese)
- 2 cups (a 6-ounce block) shredded Gruyere cheese (sub: Swiss cheese, Monterey Jack, or your favorite shredded cheese)
- 12 large eggs
- 1 cup milk (we used 2% milk, but it's your choice)

Instructions

Make It Now:

1. Cook the bacon in a large skillet over medium heat until brown and crispy, about 8 minutes.
2. Using a slotted spoon, transfer the bacon to a paper-toweled lined plate and pour off all about 2 tablespoons of grease. Set aside.
3. Turn the heat up to medium-high and add the onions and red pepper flakes. Sauté until softened, about 3-4 minutes. Stir in the peppers, kale, and garlic and cook another 1-2 minutes, until the kale has wilted, seasoning lightly with salt and pepper while it cooks. Set aside. (Freezing instructions begin here.)
4. Spray a 6-quart slow cooker insert generously with cooking spray. Layer 1 1/2 cups of the hash browns, 1/2

of the bacon, half of the veggie mixture, 1/4 cup Parmesan, and 1 cup Gruyere, and then repeat with the remaining hash browns, bacon, veggies, and cheeses.

5. In a large mixing bowl, whisk together eggs, milk, 1/4 teaspoon salt, and 1/4 teaspoon black pepper. Pour over the other ingredients in the slow cooker. (Note: The casserole can sit in the refrigerator for up to 3 days at this point.)

6. Cover and cook on Low for 4 hours, or until the center is set. Dab off any moisture from the top with a paper towel.

7. Taste and season with most salt and pepper, as needed. Serve warm.

8. Freeze for Later: Follow Steps 1-3; let the veggie mixture cool. In a large bowl, whisk together the eggs, milk, 1/4 teaspoon salt, and 1/4 teaspoon pepper. Pour the egg mixture into a gallon-sized freezer bag or container. Add in the veggies and bacon, hash browns, 1 cup of Gruyere cheese, and 1/4 cup of Parmesan cheese. Seal tightly, toss lightly to combine, and freeze. Add the remaining 1/2 cup of Gruyere and 1/4 cup of Parmesan to a small freezer bag or container and freeze along with the egg mixture.

Prep Time: 20 Minutes

Cook Time: 40 Minutes

Servings: 9

Ingredients

- 2 cups white whole wheat flour (sub: 1 cup wheat flour + 1 cup all-purpose flour)
- 1/2 cup sugar (I often use unrefined coconut sugar)
- 1 teaspoon cinnamon
- 1 teaspoon baking powder
- 1 teaspoon baking soda
- 1/2 teaspoon salt
- 2 ripe bananas
- 1 medium sweet potato, cooked and mashed (about 1 cup) (sub: pumpkin puree or butternut squash puree)
- 2 eggs
- 1 teaspoon vanilla
- 1/3 cup melted coconut oil (sub: avocado oil or melted butter)
- 1/2 cup plain Greek yogurt (sub: sour cream)

- 1/2 cup mini chocolate chips (I used carob chips, since they are low in sugar and dairy-free)

Instructions

Make It Now:

1. Preheat oven to 350°F degrees. Spray an 8×8-inch baking dish (or a 9×13 baking dish, but note the shorter cooking time) with non-stick spray.
2. In a large bowl, whisk together flour, sugar, cinnamon, baking powder, baking soda, and salt. Set aside.
3. In a blender, combine the bananas, sweet potato, eggs, vanilla, coconut oil, and yogurt. Blend until smooth. (If needed, add just a splash of milk to help the blender get moving.)
4. Using a spatula to clean out the blender, add the wet ingredients to the dry ingredients. Stir gently with a spoon just until combined (do not over-mix). Batter will be thick. Fold in the chocolate chips.
5. Spoon batter into prepared pan and spread evenly using a spatula.
6. Bake for about 35-40 minutes (for a 9×12, bake 25-28 minutes). It's done when a toothpick inserted in center of cake comes out clean. Cool completely.

7. Freeze for Later: Bake breakfast cake just until done. Cool completely. Either cover the baking dish tightly in a few layers of foil or plastic wrap or carefully lift the cake out of the baking dish and wrap in several layers of foil or plastic wrap, pressing as much air out as you can.

Prep Time: 15 Minutes

Cook Time: 35 Minutes

Servings: 9

Ingredients

Cooking spray

- 2 cups white whole wheat flour
- 1 teaspoon baking powder
- 1 teaspoon baking soda
- 1 1/2 teaspoons ground cinnamon
- 1/2 teaspoon salt
- 1/3 cup avocado oil (sub: melted, cooled coconut oil)
- 2 large eggs
- 1/2 cup sugar (I use coconut sugar for a little healthier alternative)
- 1/2 cup plain Greek yogurt (use vanilla Greek yogurt for more sweetness)
- 2 teaspoons vanilla extract
- 1 large overripe banana
- 1 medium zucchini, diced (about 2 1/2 cups diced zucchini)

- 1/2 cup mini chocolate chips

Instructions

Make It Now:

1. Prep: Preheat the oven to 350°F degrees. Spray a 9×9 inch or 8×8 inch baking dish with cooking spray.
2. Dry Ingredients: In a large bowl, whisk together flour, baking soda, cinnamon, and salt. Set aside.
3. Wet Ingredients: Add the oil, eggs, sugar, yogurt, vanilla, banana, and zucchini to a high-powered blender. Secure the lid and blend until smooth.
4. Combine: Add the wet ingredients to the dry ones and stir just until it starts to come together (do not stir a lot here). Add the chocolate chips and stir until fully combined, being careful not to overmix.
5. Bake: Pour batter into the dish. Bake for 30-35 minutes for a 9×9 inch pan or 40-45 minutes for 8×8 inch pan, or until a toothpick inserted in center of cake comes out mostly clean. Place on a cooling rack and let cool for at least 10 minutes.
6. Freeze for Later: Bake the cake just until done. Cool completely. Either cover the baking dish tightly in a few layers of foil or plastic wrap or carefully lift the cake out

of the baking dish and wrap in several layers of foil or plastic wrap, pressing as much air out as you can. Label and freeze.

10. Blueberry Crumble Cake

Prep Time: 15 Minutes

Cook Time: 40 Minutes

Servings: 10

Ingredients

Crumble Topping:

- 5 tablespoons flour
- 1/2 cup granulated sugar
- 1 teaspoon ground cinnamon
- 1 teaspoon grated lemon zest
- Pinch of salt
- 4 tablespoons unsalted butter

Cake:

- 1 3/4 cups white whole wheat flour (sub: all-purpose flour)
- 1/4 cup ground flax seed (sub: flour)
- 2 teaspoons baking powder
- 1/2 teaspoon table salt
- 4 tablespoons unsalted butter, softened
- 3/4 cup sugar

- 1 large egg

- 1 teaspoon vanilla extract

- 1 pint (2 cups) blueberries – I used frozen and tossed them in flour to keep them from sinking

- 1/2 cup whole milk

- Confectioners' sugar, for dusting (optional)

Instructions

1. Heat oven to 375°F. Butter a 9×9 inch baking dish.

2. Prepare the crumble topping by mixing the flour, sugar, cinnamon, lemon zest and salt, then cutting the butter in with a pastry blender, fork or your fingertips until the mixture resembles coarse crumbs. Set aside.

3. In a medium mixing bowl whisk together flour, flax seed, baking powder, and salt until combined. In a large bowl, beat butter and sugar until light and fluffy. Add egg, vanilla, and milk and beat until combined. Slowly add in the dry ingredients until everything is combined. The batter will be very stiff. Lastly, gently fold the blueberries into cake batter until they are evenly distributed.

4. Scoop cake batter into prepared pan and smooth so that it is flat. Sprinkle the crumble topping on top of

the batter. Bake in heated oven for 40 minutes, or until a toothpick inserted into the middle of the cake comes out batter-free. Let the cake cool a bit before removing it from the dish. Dust with confectioners' sugar, if using.

11. Hash Brown Casserole

Prep Time: 15 Minutes

Cook Time: 50 Minutes

Servings: 6

Ingredients

- 1 teaspoon avocado oil or olive oil
- 1 pound all-natural ground pork sausage or turkey sausage
- 3 cups refrigerated or thawed frozen shredded hash browns
- 1 1/2 cups shredded cheddar cheese (DF option: Omit the cheese.)
- 6 large eggs
- 1/2 cup milk (DF option: Use unsweetened, plain almond milk or oat milk.)
- 1/4 teaspoon salt, plus more to taste
- 1/4 teaspoon ground black pepper, plus more to taste
- Optional toppings: hot sauce, salsa, ketchup, freshly chopped tomatoes, and avocado

- You'll need to mostly thaw your frozen hash browns before putting together this casserole. Do this overnight in fridge or using your microwaves defrost setting? Dab off any excess moisture paper towel.

Instructions

Make It Now:

1. Preheat the oven to 350°F.

2. Heat the oil in a medium-sized skillet over medium-high heat. Once the oil is shimmery, add the sausage and cook until browned and cooked through, breaking it up as it cooks. Transfer the sausage to a paper towel–lined plate to drain and set aside.

3. Generously spray an 8×8-inch casserole dish with cooking spray. Layer 1 1/2 cups of the hash browns, half the sausage, and 3/4 cup of the cheese in the dish, then repeat with the remaining hash browns, sausage, and cheese.

4. In a large bowl, whisk together the eggs, milk, salt, and pepper. Pour over the ingredients in the dish. (Freezing instructions begin here.)

5. Bake, uncovered, for 50-60 minutes or until edges are bubbly, the middle is set, and top is golden. Tent with foil if the top starts to get too brown before it's done. If the casserole was still cold when you put it in or if it was previously frozen, it will likely take longer. Our tests showed that it will take about 60 minutes to bake after being frozen and thawed. This is because of the extra liquid that's released during that process.)

6. Let the casserole sit for 10 minutes before serving. Serve warm, topped with hot sauce, salsa, or ketchup, if desired. Season with more salt and pepper, if desired.

7. Freeze For Later: Skip Step 1. Follow Steps 2-4, tightly wrap the casserole in plastic wrap or foil, and freeze.

8. Prepare From Frozen: Note: You may want to have hot sauce, salsa, or ketchup on hand for serving. Thaw completely. Follow Steps 5-6, except bake for about 60 minutes or until set in the middle.

Prep Time: 10 Minutes

Cook Time: 20 Minutes

Servings: 6

Ingredients

- 6 (8-inch) whole wheat or multigrain tortillas (corn tortillas are not recommended)
- 1 cup cooked brown rice
- 1 cup black or kidney beans, cooked or canned (drained and rinsed)
- 1 cup corn, frozen or canned (drained)
- 1/2 cup salsa (your favorite kind)
- 1 cup shredded cheddar cheese (how to shred your own cheese)

Instructions

Make It Now:

1. Preheat oven to 350°F.
2. Lay out the tortillas on a cutting board or clean surface. Evenly distribute the rice, beans, corn, salsa, and

cheese among each one. Roll up like a burrito, tucking in the bottom and top and rolling tightly. Wrap each burrito in foil. (Freezing instructions begin here.)

3. Bake directly on an oven rack for about 15-20 minutes, until hot all the way through.

4. Freeze For Later: Follow Steps 1 and 2. Then, place the uncooked wraps in a freezer bag and freeze for up to 3 months.

5. Prepare From Frozen: To heat from frozen, you have two options:

6. Option 1 (Oven): Cook according to Step 3, adding about 10-15 minutes on to baking time. So, the total baking time will be about 25-35 minutes.

7. Option 2 (Microwave): Remove the foil, wrap in a moist paper towel, and microwave in 30-60 second increments until heated through.

Prep Time: 10 Minutes

Cook Time: 10 Minutes

Servings: 6

Ingredients

- 6 ciabatta rolls (or 12 slices of sourdough bread)
- 6 slices Provolone cheese (or 12 slices, if you want to add 2 per panini)
- 1/2 cup Pesto
- 1/4 cup sun-dried tomatoes, finely chopped
- 1 pound all-natural deli turkey slices
- 2–3 tablespoons softened butter

Instructions

Make It Now

1. Build the Paninis: Butter the outside of both pieces of bread. Spread pesto on the inside of both pieces. To the bottom bun, add 1 slice of Provolone cheese, about 2-3 slices of turkey, and 2 teaspoons of chopped sun-dried

tomatoes. Place other bun on top. (Freezing instructions begin here.)

2. Cook the Paninis: Heat a skillet over medium-high heat. Place the sandwich (es) in the hot pan and press down with a spatula or another heavy-bottomed pan. Once the bread gets toasted on the first side and the cheese starts to melt, flip to the other side. Press the sandwich down again. Remove the sandwich from the pan once it's golden brown on the second side, after a minute or two.

Freeze For Later:

1. Follow Step 1. Wrap each sandwich in foil and place in a large freezer bag. Seal and freeze.

Prep Time: 20 Minutes

Cook Time: 10 Minutes

Servings: 6

Ingredients

- 1 cup oyster crackers
- 1/3 cup crushed multigrain crackers
- 3/4 cup grated Parmesan cheese
- 1/3 cup packed fresh parsley leaves
- 3 tablespoons chopped fresh chives
- 2 tablespoons fresh thyme leaves (or 2 teaspoons of dried thyme leaves)
- 1 tablespoon Old Bay seasoning
- 1 teaspoon garlic powder
- 3/4 cup whole wheat flour (sub: all-purpose flour)
- 2 large eggs, beaten
- Splash of water
- Salt and pepper, to taste
- About 1 cup avocado oil (or another neutral frying oil)
- 6 (4 ounce) tilapia fillets, patted dry
- Lemon wedges, for serving

Instructions

Make It Now:

1. Optional: Preheat oven to 200°F. Cover a sheet pan with foil or parchment paper and place in the oven. (This is to keep the fish hot in between batches.)

2. Add the the oyster crackers, multigrain crackers, grated Parmesan, parsley leaves, chives, thyme, Old Bay seasoning, and garlic powder to a food processor (or blender). Process until well combined into a breadcrumb-like texture.

3. Transfer the cracker mixture to a shallow dish. In another shallow dish, beat the eggs and splash of water. Finally, place the flour in a third shallow dish. Line these up near the stovetop as a breading station for the tilapia.

4. To a large skillet, add enough oil to reach a depth of ¼ inch and heat over medium-high heat until shimmery.

5. Meanwhile, season fish fillets lightly on both sides with salt and pepper. Coat the fish with the flour, shaking off any excess; coat with the egg mixture, then with the cracker crumbs.

6. Working in two batches (don't overcrowd the pan), fry the breaded fish in the skillet, turning once, until golden brown on both sides, about 5 minutes total per batch. The fish is done if it flakes easily.

7. Transfer each batch to the sheet pan in the oven to keep warm. Serve with lemon wedges.

8. Freeze For Later: Follow Steps 2-3 and 5. Place breaded filets in a gallon-sized freezer bag in a single layer. Divide layers with parchment paper. Seal tightly, squeezing out any excess air, and freeze.

Prep Time: 10 Minutes

Cook Time: 00 Minutes

Servings: 1

Ingredients

- 1/2 cup cooked black beans (drained and rinsed)
- 1/4 cup chopped bell pepper
- 1/4 cup chopped cherry tomatoes (sub: more diced peppers or a little red onion)
- 1/2 ripe avocado, chopped
- 2 tablespoons crumbled feta cheese (sub: goat cheese)
- Juice from 1/2 a lemon
- Salt, pepper, and garlic powder, to taste

Instructions

1. Combine black beans, bell pepper, tomatoes, avocado, and feta cheese in a dinner-sized bowl. Squeeze fresh lemon juice over the top and sprinkle on salt, pepper and garlic powder to taste. Stir, taste, and season as needed.

2. Eat cold or warm up for about 30-45 seconds in the microwave and stir. Serve with multigrain crackers or pita chips on the side, if you'd like. Or stir in some couscous, quinoa, or rice.

Prep Time: 45 Minutes

Cook Time: 20 Minutes

Servings: 10

Ingredients

- 2 tablespoons olive oil
- 1 large onion, diced
- 3 cloves garlic, minced
- 2 pounds ground beef (or one pound ground beef & one pound Italian sausage) Here is where you can find meat you can trust.
- 1 (28 ounce) can whole tomatoes, with juice
- 2 (14.5 ounce) cans tomato sauce
- 2 teaspoons Italian Seasoning
- 1/2 teaspoon red pepper flakes
- Salt and Pepper, to taste
- 1 pound (16 ounces) whole wheat penne pasta
- 1 tub (15 ounces) whole milk ricotta cheese
- 1 1/2 pounds (6 cups) shredded mozzarella cheese (divided)
- 1/2 cup grated Parmesan cheese

- 1 egg

Instructions

Make It Now:

1. Heat olive oil in a skillet over medium heat. Add diced onions and saute for several minutes, or until starting to soften. And garlic and cook for 30 seconds more.
2. Add ground beef and cook until browned. Drain off fat, leaving a bit behind for flavor and moisture.
3. Add tomatoes, tomato sauce, Italian seasoning, red pepper flakes, salt, and pepper. Stir and simmer for 25 to 30 minutes.
4. Remove 3 to 4 cups of the sauce to a different bowl to cool.
5. Preheat oven to 375 degrees F.
6. Begin to boil your pasta. Make sure to undercook it a tad—especially if freezing!
7. In a separate bowl, mix together the ricotta cheese, 2 cups of the grated mozzarella, Parmesan, egg, and a dash of salt and pepper.
8. Drain the pasta and rinse under cool water to stop the cooking. Pour it into the bowl with the cheese mixture and mix it together.

9. Add the cooked meat sauce that you set aside earlier and toss to combine.

10. Dump the pasta mixture into a large greased casserole dish or lasagna dish. (NOTE: I ended up using a 9×13 AND a 9×9 dish to fit all of it!) Spoon the remaining sauce over the top, then top with remaining mozzarella cheese. (Freezing instructions begin here.)

11. Bake for 20 minutes, or until bubbling. Remove from oven and let stand 5 minutes before serving. Hint: Sprinkle chopped parsley over the pasta before serving!

Prep Time: 10 Minutes

Cook Time: 8hrs 2 Minutes

Servings: 10

Ingredients

- 2 1/2 – 3 pound boneless beef chuck roast
- Kosher salt and pepper
- 1 cup beef broth (or sub chicken stock)
- 1/4 cup balsamic vinegar
- 2 tablespoons low-sodium soy sauce (Gluten-free option: Use coconut aminos or gluten-free Tamari Soy Sauce)
- 1 tablespoon honey
- 4 cloves garlic, minced
- 1/2 teaspoon red pepper flakes (increase if you want more heat)

Instructions

Make It Now:

1. Put roast beef into slow cooker and season with kosher salt and pepper on all sides.

2. In a small bowl, mix together all remaining ingredients. Pour over roast beef.

3. Slow cook on LOW for about 8 hours, or until meat easily shreds apart.

4. Using two large forks, shred the meat apart in the slow cooker.

5. Serve meat warm on top of mashed potatoes or polenta (pictured). Alternatively, serve on a bun or ciabatta roll with sauce on the side for dipping, like French Dip Sandwiches.

Freeze For Later:

1. Method 1: Uncooked

2. To Freeze: Place all ingredients together in a freezer-friendly plastic bag and freeze. To prepare, let bag thaw in refrigerator for 24 hours.

3. To Prepare: Thaw in the fridge overnight and then cook as directed.

Method 2: Fully Cooked

1. To freeze: Fully cook the meal (through Step #4). Let it cool completely. (Safety Note: Do not let the meat sit on the counter for more than 2 hours.) Store meat and

sauce in a freezer-safe container after it's cooled completely.

2. To thaw: Use one of these safe thawing methods and then warm on the stove over low heat or in the microwave.

Prep Time: 20 Minutes

Cook Time: 25 Minutes

Servings: 5

Ingredients

- 4 cups (about 1 1/2 pounds) fully-cooked chicken, shredded or cubed
- 3 cups marinara sauce (or one 24-ounce jar)
- 1/2 cup shredded or grated Parmesan cheese
- 1 1/2 cups shredded mozzarella cheese
- 1 cup Panko or regular bread crumbs (sub: gluten free bread crumbs)
- 1–2 tablespoons olive oil
- 2–4 tablespoons chopped fresh parsley (or 1 tablespoon dried parsley)
- Salt and pepper, to taste

Instructions

Make It Now:

1. Preheat oven to 350°F. Grease an 8×8 inch casserole dish with cooking spray.

2. Layer the fully-cooked chicken in the bottom. Dump in the marinara sauce and mix with the chicken. Next, top with both cheeses until all the chicken is covered.

3. In a small bowl, stir together the breadcrumbs, olive oil, fresh parsley, and a pinch of salt and pepper.

4. Sprinkle the seasoned breadcrumbs over the top. (Freezing instructions begin here.)

5. Bake for about 20-25 minutes or until golden on top and bubbling on the sides. If you want it a little more browned on top, turn on the broiler for 1-2 minutes (watch closely so it doesn't burn!). Serve "as is" or over your favorite cooked pasta or rice.

6. Freeze For Later: Follow Steps 1-4. Cover the casserole tightly with a few layers of plastic wrap and/or foil, squeezing out as much air as possible. Label and freeze for up to 3 months.

7. Prepare From Frozen: Thaw in the fridge overnight and follow Step 5. Note: If it's still slightly frozen in the middle, you'll just have to cook it longer than the recipe calls for or defrost it a bit in the microwave before baking. Cover it with foil if the top gets too brown in the oven.

Prep Time: 10 Minutes

Cook Time: 20 Minutes

Servings: 4

Ingredients

- 1 teaspoon garlic powder
- 1 teaspoon dried oregano
- 1 teaspoon ground cumin
- 1 teaspoon ground coriander
- 1/2 teaspoon ground thyme
- 1 teaspoon salt
- About 1 1/4 pounds pork tenderloin

Instructions

Make It Now:

1. Preheat the oven to 450° F.
2. In small bowl stir together garlic powder, oregano, cumin, coriander, ground thyme, and salt until well combined.

3. Place the pork tenderloin on a rimmed baking sheet. Rub the seasoning on all sides of the pork tenderloin, pressing so the seasoning adheres well. (Freezing instructions begin here.)

4. Bake until it reaches an internal temp of 140-145°F. This will take about 25 minutes, depending on the size of your pork tenderloin. Note: It will still be slightly pink inside!

5. Cover with foil and let it rest for 5-10 minutes so the juices redistribute. (The temperature will also rise another 5°F during this time.) Slice on an angle and serve.

6. Tip: Cover the sheet pan with parchment or foil for easier clean up.

7. Freeze For Later: Follow Steps 2-3. Place the seasoned pork tenderloin in a gallon-sized freezer bag, squeeze out the air and seal tightly, and freeze for up to 3 months.

8. Prepare From Frozen: Thaw the meal using one of these safe thawing methods. Place the pork on a rimmed sheet pan and follow Steps 4-5.

Prep Time: 15 Minutes

Cook Time: 20 Minutes

Servings: 15

Ingredients

- 15–20 mini wheat rolls
- 1 pound deli ham
- 7 ounces Swiss cheese slices
- 1/2 cup butter
- 1 tablespoon dijon mustard
- 1 tablespoon Worcestershire
- 1 tablespoon poppyseeds (find in spice aisle)
- 1/3 cup brown sugar

Instructions

Make It Now:

1. Preheat oven 350 degrees F.
2. Assemble the sandwiches, using 1-2 slices of folded ham and a 1/2 slice of cheese on the rolls. Place in 9×13

baking dish (or whatever size you have). Squeeze sandwiches in side by side.

3. Mix butter, mustard, Worcestershire sauce, poppy seeds and brown sugar into medium sauce pan.
4. On medium-high heat, bring sauce to a boil and then reduce heat.
5. Lightly drizzle each sandwich with the prepared sauce. (Freezing instructions begin here.)
6. Cover with foil and bake for about 20 minutes.
7. Freeze for Later: Prepare sandwiches with sauce on top in casserole dish, but do not bake. Seal tightly with a lid or wrap with plastic wrap and/or foil very well. Freeze.
8. Prepare From Frozen: Let sandwiches thaw in the refrigerator overnight. Bake according to directions in step 6.

Prep Time: 20 Minutes

Cook Time: 25 Minutes

Servings: 7

Ingredients

- Taco Seasoning Ingredients
- 1 tablespoon chili powder
- 2 teaspoon ground cumin
- 1 teaspoon salt
- 1 teaspoon black pepper
- 1/2 teaspoon garlic powder
- 1/2 teaspoon onion powder
- 1/2 teaspoon crushed red pepper flakes (or less for sensitive palates)
- 1/2 teaspoon dried oregano
- 1/2 teaspoon paprika
- Optional: 1/2 teaspoon sugar
- Taco Meat Ingredients
- 1–2 tablespoons olive oil or avocado oil
- 1 small white onion, diced (about 1 cup)

- 3–4 cloves of garlic, minced
- 2 pounds lean ground beef (sub: ground turkey)
- 1 cup beef or chicken broth
- Additional Taco Bar Ingredients (pick and choose from the ideas below)
- 12–16 taco shells (soft or hard), warmed according to package directions
- 1–2 cups chopped lettuce
- 1–2 cups diced tomatoes
- 1/2 cup diced red onion (or Pickled Red Onions)
- 2 cups shredded cheddar cheese (sub: Mexican blend or Cotija cheese)
- 1–2 avocados, diced (or Guacamole)
- 1 cup salsa (recommend: Mateo's medium salsa)
- Cilantro Lime Aioli (put in a squeeze bottle from the dollar store)
- Sour cream (sub: plain Greek yogurt)
- Fresh cilantro, chopped
- Lime wedges
- 1 (15-ounce) can black beans, rinsed and warmed (sub: pinto beans)
- Cilantro Lime Rice

Instructions

Make It Now:

1. Make Seasoning: In a small bowl, stir together taco seasoning ingredients. Set aside.

2. Saute Onion: In a large skillet, heat the oil over medium-high heat. Saute the diced onion, stirring frequently, until softened, 4 to 5 minutes. Stir in 3-4 minced garlic cloves and cook for 30 to 60 seconds more.

3. Cook Ground Meat: Add the ground beef and cook for 5-7 minutes, or until no longer pink, breaking up the meat with a wooden spoon or spatula as it browns. Drain off excess grease.

4. Season & Simmer: Sprinkle 3-4 tablespoons of taco seasoning over the meat and stir until coated. Add in 1 cup of chicken/beef/vegetable broth and bring to a simmer. Reduce the heat to medium-low and simmer, uncovered, until the mixture has reduced some, about 5 minutes.

5. Serve: Transfer cooked ground meat to a serving bowl and set out with other Mexican toppings in various shapes/sizes of bowls in an assembly line to make your homemade taco bar! Keep soft tortillas warm by wrapping in a clean dish towel.

6. Freeze for Later: Cook the meat as directed, then let the mixture cool completely. Place it in a freezer bag, seal and freeze. In separate bags, freeze about 2 cups of shredded cheese and soft tortillas along with the meat, to complete your kit.

7. Prepare For Later: Let all ingredients thaw in the refrigerator. Serve as directed.

Prep Time: 3hrs 2 Minutes

Cook Time: 16 Minutes

Servings: 23

Ingredients

- 1 1/3 cup water, lukewarm (about 110°F)
- 1 stick (1/2 cup) unsalted butter, softened
- 5 tablespoons sugar
- 1 teaspoon salt
- 1 large egg, lightly beaten
- 1 tablespoon dry active yeast
- 4 1/2 cups unbleached all-purpose flour
- Quick-rise yeast will work as well, but keep an eye on the dough as it will rise faster.

Instructions

Make It Now:

1. Add ingredients to your bread machine in the order listed. Run on the dough cycle. It should be around 90 minutes for reference.

2. Punch the dough down and then remove from bread maker.

3. Roll dough into balls (a little bigger than the size of a golf ball) and place on a greased baking sheet. Loosely cover with plastic wrap (or a thin dish towel).

4. Let dough balls rise in a warm atmosphere for 1 hour.

5. Preheat the oven to 350°F. Bake for 15-17 minutes, until starting to brown on top.

6. Freeze for Later: Bake rolls as stated in recipe. Let cool completely. Place rolls in air-tight, freezer bag or container. Freeze up to 1 month for best quality.

7. Prepare From Frozen: Let rolls thaw on the counter or in refrigerator overnight.

8. To Freeze Before Baking: Follow the steps all the way up to baking. Freeze the rolls of dough on a baking pan. Once frozen you can place them in a freezer bag. To prepare from frozen, let them thaw and rise for about 4-5 hours, then bake.

Prep Time: 15 Minutes

Cook Time: 20 Minutes

Servings: 6

Ingredients

- 1 1/2 pounds boneless, skinless chicken breasts
- 1 teaspoon salt
- 3/4 teaspoon ground black pepper
- 3 cups cooked brown rice (Shortcut: Two Uncle Ben's Ready Brown Rice 8.8 ounce packs)
- 6 tablespoons salted butter
- 4 cups broccoli florets, cut into bite-sized pieces (Shortcut: One 12 ounce package of pre-cut Hy-Vee Broccoli Florets)
- 1 1/2 cups shredded Cheddar cheese
- 12 ounces bacon, cooked and chopped into bite-sized pieces (Shortcut: Hy-Vee Fully Cooked Bacon)

Instructions

Make It Now:

1. Preheat a grill to medium-high heat or the oven to 400°F.

2. Tear off 6 pieces of heavy-duty foil that measure roughly 12×12 inches and set aside.

3. On a cutting board, dice the chicken into bite-sized pieces. Season with the salt and pepper on all sides. (If you want, you could add a little onion powder and garlic powder too, but totally optional.)

4. Assemble the Foil Packets: To each piece of foil, scoop 1/2 cup of the cooked rice and top it with 1 tablespoon of the butter. Add about 1/2 cup of chicken, 2/3 cup broccoli, 1/3 cup cheese, and about 2-3 tablespoons of the chopped bacon. Fold up the sides of the foil and seal. (Freezing instructions begin here.)

5. Cook the Foil Packets: You have two options for cooking the foil packs. Either place the foil packs directly on the grill (do not close the lid) or in the oven and cook for 20-25 minutes. (The chicken is done when a thermometer inserted in the chicken registers 165°F or no longer is pink in the middle. The broccoli should be tender, as well.)

6. Remove the foil packs from the heat (using tongs) and let stand for about 5 minutes. Carefully open each pack to release the steam and enjoy!

7. Freeze For Later: Follow Steps 2-4. Place the foil packets in a large freezer bag or container. Seal and freeze.

8. Prepare From Frozen: Thaw completely in the refrigerator. Follow Step 1 and then Steps 5-6.

Prep Time: 20 Minutes

Cook Time: 25 Minutes

Servings: 6

Ingredients

- 4 cups (about 1 1/2 pounds) fully-cooked chicken, shredded or cubed
- 3 cups marinara sauce (or one 24-ounce jar)
- 1/2 cup shredded or grated Parmesan cheese
- 1 1/2 cups shredded mozzarella cheese
- 1 cup Panko or regular bread crumbs (sub: gluten free bread crumbs)
- 1–2 tablespoons olive oil
- 2–4 tablespoons chopped fresh parsley (or 1 tablespoon dried parsley)
- Salt and pepper, to taste

Instructions

Make It Now:

1. Preheat oven to 350°F. Grease an 8×8 inch casserole dish with cooking spray.

2. Layer the fully-cooked chicken in the bottom. Dump in the marinara sauce and mix with the chicken. Next, top with both cheeses until all the chicken is covered.

3. In a small bowl, stir together the breadcrumbs, olive oil, fresh parsley, and a pinch of salt and pepper.

4. Sprinkle the seasoned breadcrumbs over the top. (Freezing instructions begin here.)

5. Bake for about 20-25 minutes or until golden on top and bubbling on the sides. If you want it a little more browned on top, turn on the broiler for 1-2 minutes (watch closely so it doesn't burn!). Serve "as is" or over your favorite cooked pasta or rice.

6. Freeze For Later: Follow Steps 1-4. Cover the casserole tightly with a few layers of plastic wrap and/or foil, squeezing out as much air as possible. Label and freeze for up to 3 months.

7. Prepare From Frozen: Thaw in the fridge overnight and follow Step 5. Note: If it's still slightly frozen in the middle, you'll just have to cook it longer than the recipe calls for or defrost it a bit in the microwave before baking. Cover it with foil if the top gets too brown in the oven.

Prep Time: 20 Minutes

Cook Time: 20 Minutes

Servings: 25

Ingredients

- 1/2 cup whole wheat bread crumbs (here's how to make your own)
- 1/2 cup grated Parmesan cheese
- 2 tablespoons finely chopped fresh parsley
- 2 tablespoons minced chives
- 1/2 cup finely shredded carrot
- 1/2 cup finely shredded zucchini (squeeze out the excess moisture)
- 1 large egg, beaten
- 3 tablespoons ketchup (preferably organic)
- 1 1/2 pounds lean ground beef (sub: ground turkey)
- 1 teaspoon salt
- 1/2 teaspoon pepper
- 1/2 teaspoon garlic powder
- After retesting, this recipe was updated on 3/2/23. Changes are in the notes below.

Instructions

Make It Now:

1. Prep: Preheat oven to 400°F. Cover a rimmed sheet pan with parchment paper or foil for easy clean-up. Optional: Place a cooking rack on top of the sheet pan to let the fat drip below.

2. Combine Meat Mixture: In a large bowl, use a fork to stir together the breadcrumbs, grated Parmesan, parsley, chives, carrot, zucchini, beaten egg, and ketchup. Add in the ground beef by pinches (to break it up a bit) and then sprinkle the salt, pepper, and garlic powder evenly over the top of the beef. Use your hands to combine the mixture but do not over mix.

3. Roll Meatballs: Using a heaping tablespoon of mixture per meatball, roll into 1 1/2 inch meatballs. Place them on the sheet pan (either directly on it or on top of the rack), leaving a little room between each one.

4. Bake in the Oven: Bake for 15-18 minutes or until cooked through. (If your meatballs are on a rack, they may take a few extra minutes.) Cut one open and make sure there is no pink in the middle to assure doneness. Internal temp should be 160°F.

5. Serve: Serve with Marinara Sauce or Pesto over pasta or on Meatball Subs.

Freeze For Later:

1. Option 1 (Uncooked Meatballs): Follow steps 1-3. Place sheet pan of meatballs in the freezer until frozen and then place the frozen meatballs in a freezer bag. Seal and freeze.

2. Option 2 (Fully Cooked Meatballs): Follow steps 1-4. Let cool completely. Freeze the cooked meatballs in a freezer bag or container. Tip: Freeze the meatballs in marinara sauce to help keep them moist.

Prep Time: 5 Minutes

Cook Time: 5 Minutes

Servings: 4

Ingredients

- 1/4 cup olive oil
- 3 tablespoons fresh lemon juice (juice of about 1 1/2 lemons)
- 1 teaspoon of minced garlic (2–3 garlic cloves, minced)
- 1 teaspoon salt
- 1/4 teaspoon freshly ground black pepper
- 1/8 teaspoon red pepper flakes
- 1/2 teaspoon dried oregano
- 1/2 teaspoon dried basil
- 1 pound raw deveined large (16/20 count) shrimp (peeled or shell on)
- Fresh parsley, chopped, for garnish
- Lemon wedges, for garnish
- Crumbled feta cheese, for garnish (optional)

Instructions

Make It Now:

1. In a medium bowl, combine all marinade ingredients, from olive oil through dried basil.
2. Pat dry the shrimp with paper towels. Then add to the marinade and toss. Set in the refrigerator for 30 minutes to marinate. Stir occasionally.
3. Preheat oven broiler. Line a baking sheet with foil for easy cleanup.
4. Optional: Thread four or five shrimp on each skewer. Set shrimp on baking sheet. Discard the rest of the marinade (or boil marinade and use as sauce per serving instructions below.)
5. Broil shrimp for 2 minutes on the first side and then flip the shrimp. Broil for another 2 minutes on the second side. Shrimp is done when it is pink. Do not overcook.
6. Garnish shrimp with some minced parsley, a squeeze of lemon, and some crumbled feta. Serve warm or at room temperature.

Prep Time: 5 Minutes

Cook Time: 8 Minutes

Servings: 4

Ingredients

- 8 ounces dried pasta (i.e. egg noodles, linguine, thin spaghetti, etc)
- 2 tablespoons salted butter
- 1/4 teaspoon garlic salt
- 2 tablespoons grated Parmesan cheese
- Salt and pepper, to taste

Instructions

1. Bring a medium-sized pot of salted water to a boil over high heat. Add the pasta. Cook according to the pasta instructions.
2. Drain the pasta and return it to the pot.
3. Add in the butter and stir it until it melts in.
4. Add in the garlic salt and Parmesan cheese. Taste and add salt and pepper as needed.

Prep Time: 10 Minutes

Cook Time: 8hrs 2 Minutes

Servings: 6

Ingredients

- 1 cup beef broth
- 1/4 cup balsamic vinegar
- 2 tablespoons soy sauce (Gluten-free: Use coconut aminos or gluten-free Tamari Soy Sauce)
- 1 tablespoon honey
- 4 cloves garlic, minced (2 teaspoons pre-minced garlic)
- 1/2 teaspoon red pepper flakes (increase if you want more heat)
- 2 teaspoons salt, plus more to taste
- 1/2 teaspoon black pepper, plus more to taste
- 5 lbs bone-in English-style beef short ribs, trimmed of excess fat and cut crosswise into 2-inch pieces
- 2 tablespoons cornstarch (optional, but recommended)
- Fresh parsley, chopped (as garnish)
- Ask your butcher to do this for you! You might even want to call ahead.

Instructions

Make It Now:

1. Prep Marinade: In a small mixing bowl, whisk together the beef broth, vinegar, soy sauce, honey, garlic, red pepper flakes, salt, and black pepper.
2. Cook: Place the ribs in the crockpot. Pour the marinade over the top and stir to coat the ribs. Cover and cook on LOW for 8 to 10 hours. Use tongs to transfer the ribs to a serving platter.
3. Thicken Sauce: Optional, but recommended: Carefully pour or ladle the remaining juices from the crockpot into a medium saucepan. In a small bowl, stir together the cornstarch and 2 tablespoons water until smooth. Whisk this into the sauce and bring to a boil. Cook, whisking regularly, until thickened, about 2-3 minutes.
4. Serve: Drizzle some of the sauce over the ribs and garnish with chopped parsley. Serve warm with extra sauce on the side. Tip: These are delicious served over warm mashed potatoes or polenta.

To Freeze For Later:

1. Follow Step 1. Place the ribs and sauce in either a 2-gallon freezer bag or two, 1-gallon freezer bags. Seal tightly and freeze.

Prepare From Frozen:

2. You will need cornstarch and parsley on hand to complete this meal. Thaw in the refrigerator completely. Follow Steps 2-4.

Prep Time: 20 Minutes

Cook Time: 30 Minutes

Servings: 3

Ingredients

- 1 batch of whole wheat pizza dough (or 1 large pizza dough ball for a 16-inch pizza from a local pizzeria)
- 1 egg
- 2 1/2 cups store-bought or homemade pizza sauce, divided
- 3–4 ounces uncured pepperoni (sub: turkey pepperoni or deli ham slices)
- 1 pound ground Italian pork or turkey sausage, fully cooked, crumbled, and drained (sub: 2 cups thinly sliced mushrooms and/or diced bell peppers)
- 3 cups shredded mozzarella shredded cheese
- 2 tablespoons grated Parmesan cheese, plus more for optional topping
- 1 teaspoon Italian seasoning, plus more for optional topping

- 1/4 teaspoon garlic powder, plus more for optional topping

Instructions

3. Prepare: Preheat the oven to 375°F. Cover one or two large baking sheets with parchment paper. In a small bowl, whisk together the egg and 1 tablespoon water. Set aside.

4. Roll out Dough: Divide the pizza dough in half. On a lightly floured surface, roll out one of the dough balls into a large rectangle, about 11×15 inches. Make sure a long edge is closest to you for easy rolling later. (Watch our video to see how.)

5. Toppings: Spread 1/4 cup of pizza sauce over the dough, leaving a 1 1/2 inch border on the long side that's away from you. Leave at least 1/2 inch border on all other sides. Over the sauce, evenly distribute half the pepperoni, half the sausage (about 1 cup), and 1 1/2 cups mozzarella cheese. Sprinkle 1 tablespoon grated Parmesan cheese, 1/4 teaspoon Italian seasoning, and 1/8 teaspoon garlic powder over the top.

6. Roll Stromboli: Using a pastry brush, paint the short borders and long border that's farthest from you with

egg wash. Starting with the long end that's close to you, slowly roll up the dough into a cylinder, pulling in the edges along the way to seal. (Watch our video to see how.)

7. Finish the Outside: Place the stromboli seam-side down on the prepared baking sheet. Using a pastry brush, brush the top and sides of the stromboli with egg wash. Optional: Sprinkle the top with a little Italian seasoning, garlic powder, and grated Parmesan cheese, to your preference. Cut 4 diagonal 1-inch slits across the top to allow steam to release.

8. Prep 2nd Stromboli: Repeat Steps 2-5 and place the second stromboli on the second baking sheet or freeze it for later using the instructions below.

9. Cook: Bake until golden brown, about 25-30 minutes. If baking two at a time, rotate the pans halfway through baking. Remove from the oven and let stand for 10 minutes.

10. Serve: Warm the remaining pizza sauce in a pot over medium-low heat or in the microwave (be sure to cover it to avoid splatters). Using a serrated knife, slice the stromboli into 1/2-inch slices and serve with ramekins of warm pizza sauce for dipping.

Prep Time: 00 Minutes

Cook Time: 25 Minutes

Servings: 6

Ingredients

- 1/4 cup avocado oil (sub: olive oil)
- Zest of 2 limes (reserve the limes for juicing at the end)
- 1 1/2 teaspoons cumin
- 1 1/2 teaspoons chili powder
- 1 teaspoon oregano, crushed in hand
- 1 teaspoon salt, plus more to taste
- 1/2 teaspoon ground black pepper, plus more to taste
- 1/2 teaspoon garlic powder (sub: 1 1/2 teaspoon minced garlic)
- Pinch of red pepper flakes

Other Fajita Ingredients:

- 3/4 lbs tender steak, sliced across the grain into thin strips (recommended: ribeye, sirloin, culotte) (sub: chicken breasts)

- 3/4 lbs boneless, skinless chicken breasts, cut in half lengthwise and sliced across the grain into thin strips (sub: steak)
- 3 tablespoons avocado oil or olive oil
- 2–3 bell peppers, sliced 1/4-inch thick (your choice of colors)
- 1 large yellow or red onion, sliced 1/4-inch thick
- 1/2 teaspoon sugar
- 10–12 fajita-size flour tortillas (GF option: corn tortillas or gluten-free tortillas)
- Optional Toppings: lime wedges, chopped cilantro, salsa, guacamole or avocado chunks, and sour cream (DF option: omit sour cream)

Instructions

Make It Now:

1. Make the Marinade: Open 2 gallon-sized freezer bags. To each one, add the following:
1. 2 tablespoons oil
2. Zest of 1 lime (about 1 1/2 teaspoons)
3. 3/4 teaspoon cumin
4. 3/4 teaspoon chili powder
5. 1/2 teaspoon oregano, crushed in hand

6. 1/2 teaspoon salt

7. 1/4 teaspoon pepper

8. 1/4 teaspoon garlic powder

9. Small pinch of red pepper flakes

10. Use your hands to massage the bags from the bottom and combine the marinade. Then, add the steak to one bag and the chicken to the other (Do Not Add Them To The Same Bag), seal, and toss until the meat is evenly coated. (Freezing instructions begin here.)

2. Marinate the Chicken and Steak: Place the steak and chicken bags in the refrigerator to marinate for at least 1 hour and up to 24 hours, turning and/or massaging occasionally.

3. Stir Fry the Veggies: In a large skillet, heat 2 tablespoons oil over medium high heat until shimmery. Carefully add the peppers and onions to the hot pan and saute until softened and charred, 5-7 minutes for fresh veggies or 7-9 minutes for frozen veggies. Season lightly with salt and pepper and the sugar (a key ingredient!) as they cook. Remove to a platter.

4. Stir Fry the Chicken and Steak: Add 1 tablespoon of oil to the pan. Once it's shimmery, saute the steak in one batch until brown on all sides, about 3 minutes. Then, saute the chicken in second batch, about 4-5 minutes

(make sure there's no pinker on any of the chicken!). Remove to the serving platter with the veggies.

5. Serve: Squeeze half a lime over all the meat and veggies. Top with chopped cilantro, if desired. Warm the tortillas according to package directions. Serve the meat and veggies on the tortillas with lime wedges and your favorite Tex-Mex toppings.

Freeze For Later:

1. Follow Step 1. Freeze the marinated steak and chicken bags, alongside frozen peppers and onions. Two options for the frozen peppers and onions: 1) Buy a 20-22 ounce bag of frozen sliced peppers and onions, or 2) line up the fresh onion and pepper slices in a single layer on a sheet pan. Place in the freezer until solid and then put frozen veggies in a freezer bag.

Prepare From Frozen:

2. Thaw the bags of steak and chicken using one of these safe methods, but do NOT thaw the peppers and onions. Follow Steps 3-5.

www.ingramcontent.com/pod-product-compliance
Lightning Source LLC
Chambersburg PA
CBHW061002260726
48661CB00005B/2006